EAR CANDLING

THE ESSENTIAL GUIDE AND OVERVIEW OF THE PRACTICE

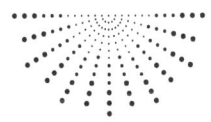

SANDRA HOPE

© Copyright 2019 - All rights reserved.

The content contained within this book may not be reproduced, duplicated or transmitted without direct written permission from the author or the publisher.

Under no circumstances will any blame or legal responsibility be held against the publisher, or author, for any damages, reparation, or monetary loss due to the information contained within this book. Either directly or indirectly.

ISBN: 9781086314533

Legal Notice:

This book is copyright protected. This book is only for personal use. You cannot amend, distribute, sell, use, quote or paraphrase any part, or the content within this book, without the consent of the author or publisher.

Disclaimer Notice:

Please note the information contained within this document is for educational and entertainment purposes only. All effort has been executed to present accurate, up to date, and reliable, complete information. No warranties of any kind are declared or implied. Readers acknowledge that the author is not engaging in the rendering of legal, financial, medical or professional advice. The content within this book has been derived from various sources. Please consult a licensed professional before attempting any techniques outlined in this book.

By reading this document, the reader agrees that under no circumstances is the author responsible for any losses, direct or indirect, which are incurred as a result of the use of information contained within this document, including, but not limited to, — errors, omissions, or inaccuracies.

CONTENTS

Foreword v
Introduction ix

1. What is Ear Candling 1
2. How Does it Work? 5
3. Sinus Issues & The Ears 11
4. Sore Throats & The Ears 17
5. Spirituality 23
6. Best Practices 29
7. Doctoral Theories 35
8. Other Ways of Natural Ear Cleaning 39

Afterword 45
Thank You 47
Resources Page 49

FOREWORD

Hi there,

I wanted to take a little of time to introduce myself and explain why I wrote this book, but first...

... I would like to sincerely thank you for purchasing this book. It truly means a lot.

Now who am I? My name is Sandra and I have been interested in alternative health and medicine for a large portion of my life.

Luckily, I do not have an inspiring story to share with you about how I was gravely ill and nursed myself back to health...

... but,

... I have experienced enough to know that modern medicine does not have all the answers. There are many natural remedies that work better than whatever chemical pills big Pharma is prescribing nowadays. I believe we came from nature and that is also where the things that heal us come from.

In my work I like to try to take an unbiased look at the issues. More often than not things are not as simple as good and bad.

Anyway...

Thanks again and enjoy the read!

Nature itself is the best physician...

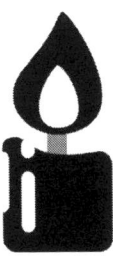

-Hippocrates-

INTRODUCTION

An art form that soothes the mind, body and soul.

Ear Candling is a procedure that goes back many, many years. The art dates back to biblical times, when practitioners took hollow reeds from swamps to use as candles. Overtime, candling continued to develop and has been passed down for generations by Native American, African, European and Oriental cultures.

Today, the procedure has once again become increasingly popular. It is a soothing and relaxing treatment that can provide a lot of health benefits. Although it is a controversial practice many find it to be incredibly calming to their head and ears.

Candling is said to be particularly great for individuals suffering from clogged ears and congestion in the head area. Clogged ears can have strong negative effects that lead to earaches, sore throats and headaches. Many people have found a solution through candling. The practice is painless, cleansing and soothing.

In this book I aim to shine a light on the art and provide a guide to best practices surrounding it. I will also examine the controversial aspects of candling, and consider some unbiased insights.

The greatest medicine of all is to teach people how not to need it.

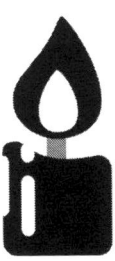

-Hippocrates-

1
WHAT IS EAR CANDLING

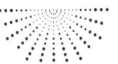

*E*ar candling is an alternative medicine procedure that claims to improve health and restore head balance. This is accomplished with the use of a hollow candle. One end of the candle is placed in a patient's ear, and the other end is lit. The process creates a very calming sound reminiscent of the ocean, and some practitioners claim it draws impurities out of the ear.

Ear candling has become a very controversial topic. Some medical research has found candling to be ineffective. Studies show that the procedure does not remove earwax, and some health physicians find it to be dangerous. There is also much debate about the history of the practice. Tibet, China, Egypt and a Native American tribe (*Hopi tribe*) have all been mentioned as places where the practice may have originated. There continue to be many questions, and few answers.

Although there is much controversy surrounding the practice, many claim to experience tremendous benefits from candling. Patients mention that the heat energy from the candle along with the sound relieves discomfort and pain. It is a gentle procedure that is much less invasive than other ear treatments like syringing. Treatments commonly take around 30 minutes and are usually followed with an easing face massage. The massage helps drain sinuses and reinforces good blood flow.

The candles used for candling are often made out of cotton or linen and infused with various aromas. This provides aromatherapy effects that encourage relaxation and reduced stress. As the candle burns the cotton vaporizes, and it is believed that impurities are pulled out of the ear through a "chimney effect". Debris are collected at the bottom of the candle or burned away.

There are many people who claim that candling helps with recovery from a flu or when you are suffering from head congestion. It may help ease the symptoms as your sinuses and ears are connected. Alleviating pressure in your ears can help get rid of stuffiness, dizziness and pain. Candling can potentially also assist with relaxing your mind and de-stressing. The procedure involves natural scents and oils that can be related back to aromatherapy. Some patients say they reach an almost meditational state during candling.

A candle loses nothing by lighting another candle...

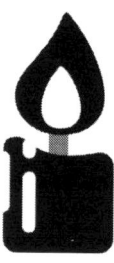

-James Keller-

2

HOW DOES IT WORK?

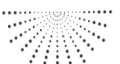

*I*t is believed that there is a constant flow of energy running through our bodies. When we are healthy, fit and just feeling great this energy can power us forward. It is a great state of flow to be in. If the body is under tension however, this flow of energy decreases. Tension, congestions or infections block the flow of the energy inside of us and allows for symptoms to appear in the body. It is said that this can be experienced through stuffiness, headaches and other annoying ailments. Below we will take a deeper look at how candling can assist our wellbeing.

The Concept

As mentioned above, it is believed that we have energy

running throughout our bodies. It keeps one balanced and in a positive flow state. This is especially important when it comes to ones head. If you experience any blockages in the head area, be it through a simple headache or a full on migraine, you simply cannot function properly. The blockage can evolve to having experiencing dizziness, throat aches, allergies and swelling. Simply put, any blockages in the head area are intensely uncomfortable and slow down even the best of us.

Remove earwax?

The concept of candling has very little to do with removing ear wax and clearing up blockages in this way. In fact, candling is not an effective way of removing ear wax at all. Contrary to what most people believe, earwax is crucial to our wellbeing. We need it for protection from dust or dirt sliding into our ears. It is also an extra barrier against harsh sounds that can damage our sensitive ear drums.

Too much earwax can become problematic. This buildup occurs when we are consistently in areas that are too noisy and have too much pollution or dust. With extreme wax buildup it is best to visit an ear specialist or physician.

. . .

The Process

During ear candling the unlit open end of a candle is placed in a persons ear. The other side gets lit has carries a small, controlled flame. Similarly to what happens inside a chimney, the burning of the candle draws from the unlit end. This very light pulling process along with the warmth the flame generates are said to relax the body. Many find that this gives back power to the body to assist in the healing process. Once relaxed and in a good flowing state that body can begin to proceed with healing itself. It can clear blockages and allow energy to run smoothly through the body again. The whole head area clears up, and the body can stabilize.

Outside and around the ear there are pressure points. These points are similar to what we commonly find in feet and hand reflexology. Stimulating these points can release tension and allow us to ease stress. This is why when we experience a headache we naturally look to massage the temples of our head. During ear candling we work around the ear space and look to activate the reflex points in the area. This happens through the heat of the candle, aromas and touch. The pressure points can eventually relax and so the body gets assisted with healing itself naturally.

. . .

Ear Candling is a spiritual therapy. The candle not only provides warmth to ease aches, it also represents as a symbol for burning away any mental blockages like fear or guilt. After the candling process an individual is free from these mental stresses holding them back. A weight is lifted, as you are cleaned from inner struggles and unwanted emotions.

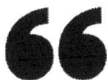

Look at how a single candle can both defy and define the darkness...

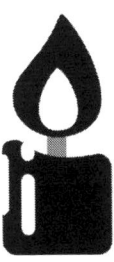

-Anne Frank-

3

SINUS ISSUES & THE EARS

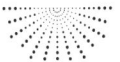

*I*ndividuals with sinus issues and allergies like hay fever experience some of the most unbearable symptoms. You are drowsy and have no energy. Your ears and nose are clogged and running, somehow at the same time. You simply don't feel comfortable in your own skin.

Many recommend putting aside any reservations you may have in regards to ear candling and trying it out to deal with sinus issues. In this chapter we will explore the connection between sinus problems and our ears.

The Connection

Sinus infections or 'sinusitis' is when someone experiences inflammation of the mucous membrane. Having facial pain, a plugged nose, fever, headaches, a sore throat and a cough are all symptoms. As our bodies are formed by a series of connections, it is common for issues to be linked. If you are suffering from a sinus infection, you are more susceptible to having ear issues.

Ear Infections

As mentioned above our bodies are a series of connections. This means our nasal area, cheekbones and ears are all connected. There is a main connector among these three elements called the 'auditory tube'. It connects the sinuses and has important health functions that keep us balanced. Unfortunately, this tube also allows infections to spread more easily throughout our heads. If water enters the tube, it can not get drained. This makes it very susceptible to bacterial and fungus growth which lead to ear infections.

Sinus Infections

Sinus infections are generally caused by a cold or hay fever. It occurs when there is an infection in the 'sinus cavities'. The sinus areas most affected by an infection range from just above your nostrils to your eyebrows. That whole area can get congested and stuffy. Your body will react by producing excessive mucus and try to get rid of bacteria or dirt. When the mucus gets build up to a point where it can no longer drain out properly, there is a high risk for infection. The sinus area will continue to get irritated and swell. This then evolves into headaches and ear issues as congestion continues to build up.

Simple things like yawning, coughing, sneezing and even chewing allow congestion to move around from the sinuses to the ears. The connections in our heads make it simple for infections to spread. All the actions mentioned above, like sneezing for example, forces air to try escape through all outlets. This includes the ears and so infections continue to disperse.

Ear Candling and other Solutions

Some experts suggest candling as a solution along with cleansing the sinus cavities two times a day (In the morning and evenings). The cleaning can be completed with the help of a simple saline solution. This clears out congestion and lowers swelling. Cleansing the sinus cavities consistently will restore your body's natural balance in the head area and allow for the sinuses to function smoothly.

It is also recommended to keep the ear canals clean. This

will prevent bacteria from building up and stop sinus ear issues. You must be very careful with placing cotton tipped cleaners in your ears, but they can help remove excessive dirt.

A last great tip when suffering from sinus & ear related issues is practicing general cleanliness. Make sure you wash your hands often and keep them clean. Also try to ensure that the areas you frequent are clean. Change your bedsheets and pillow sheets often. This will go a long way in making sure you are free from infections and can stay as healthy as possible.

If after following the tips mentioned above you continue to experience issues regularly, I recommend consulting a specialist. They will be able to prescribe some natural antihistamines and provide further medical help.

There are two ways of spreading light: to be the candle or the mirror that reflects it...

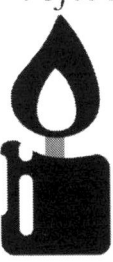

-Edith Wharton-

4

SORE THROATS & THE EARS

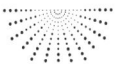

*N*ow that we understand all the connections with the sinus areas and ears, we can explore the connection between our throats and ears. Just as everyone has likely experienced a headache or stuffed nose, it is likely you have had a sore throat before. It is uncomfortable and depending on severity can make it painful to swallow.

Candling is said to help with many ailments. It is an extremely relaxing treatment. Many physicians say there is however, no evidence to support candling as a relevant treatment. In this chapter I will explore the connection between the ears and throat and look into the issues.

The Connection

Candling experts say that during a procedure the ear canals are able to release pressure and open up. This in turn, allows the body to naturally carry off an infection. So how does this affect one's throat?

A sore throat happens when there is an inflammation in the throat area. It is usually accompanied by a painful 'scratching' sensation. It can make it difficult to swallow and eat. The inflammation in the throat is caused by bacterial, fungal or viral infections. Pollutants or chemical substances may also cause a throat ache. Cleanliness is again a key point. If you are in contact with too much dust or other irritants, you are at a greater risk of getting a sore throat. Anywhere viruses or bacteria can thrive will cause health risks.

It is common for a sore throat to accompany a cold, or vice versa. As we mentioned in the previous chapter, the congestion this causes may cause your ears to get blocked. A great way to fight these illnesses and symptoms is with the help of antibiotics. They will be no help however, if it comes from a viral infection.

The connections in our body make it common for people to suffer from throat aches and ear issues at the same time. Doctoral analysis' have shown the direct relationship between the throat and ears. The auditory tube (Eustachian) connects the middle ear to the top, back of the throat. The main job of this tube is to keep fluids out of the middle ear. Because of this intricate connection between the throat and ear they can function as one unit. The main downside however is that if there is an issue with one, the other can also suffer.

A throat ache can cause the auditory tube to swell. The swelling in turn creates a lot of pressure throughout the tube which leads all the way up to the middle ear. This can be painful and now the individual has not only a sore throat, but also an ear ache.

Sore throats are usually at the end of a chain reaction. In most cases it is the body's reaction to a deeper issue. The true issue is more likely a fever, bad cough or an upper respiratory infection. By itself, a throat ache is not a major issue. It of course causes plenty of discomfort, and therefore people look to consult a doctor.

Ear, Nose & Throat

There are a variety of intricate connections between the throat, nose and ears. They can work well together as a unit but if one system suffers it can easily spread on to all three. If there is an infection or inflammation in one area, it is very likely for all parts to be impacted. A common example is the sinuses located in our nose, which are very closely connected to our throat and ears. If we suffer from a sinus infection, we feel terrible because our entire heads are under pressure. We have a blocked nose, clogged ears and a sore throat.

Candling experts advocate a procedure with them to help offer relief. The warmth and aromas gently and naturally release pressures in the head. The intricate connections and working together of the ears, nose and throat also make it easier to provide some relief. Doctors will further prescribe medicines that can assist in the healing process. In extreme cases antibiotics and syrups will help a lot with fighting illnesses.

All the darkness in the world can't put out the light of one candle...

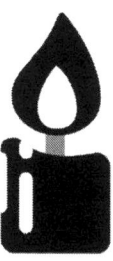

-Confucius-

5
SPIRITUALITY

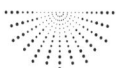

When further exploring the history of ear candling, we can see it was something practiced all over the world. While we are not sure about it always being a healing practice, we are quite sure candling was utilized for spiritual reasons.

Paintings, temple walls and pottery all depict the art being practiced. An individual sitting with a type of 'candle' in their ear. These images have been traced back to the Ancient Egyptians, Chinese and Phoenicians. We can estimate that it was used as a way to reach the spirit world.

We should note that candling was a practice reserved only for a "high-class" individual. Royalty, priests and the wealthy of the time would be allowed to make contact with the spirit world. In this chapter we will further explore candling and spiritual connection.

Native American Candling Spirituality

Some of the most discussed ear candling practices stem from the Native Americans. In their stories and music it becomes clear that they used candling for healing, along with spiritual work. Old spiritual and tribe leaders would use the practice for vision quests.

In the north-west region of North America the natives would use a clay cone as a candle. They would place herbs inside the cone that would slowly burn. The thick smoke from the cone and herbs is said to have coiled down into the ear and withdraw impurities. Depending on tribe it would also be a way of starting a vision quest.

More towards the south in what is today recognized as Mexico Natives would use old rolled up paper to make their cones. The paper was again filled up with herbs that slowly burned. Once lit the cone would be used for candling and spiritual work.

. . .

Spirituality Today

Nowadays in some parts of Europe candling is intertwined as a study of natural healing. Some doctors go through an internship or study that uses ear candling. In the United States, the practice is much more of a home remedy that gets passed down generationally.

There are several reasons why ear candling is used to explore spirituality. It is believed that it enhances extrasensory perception, more commonly known as a sixth sense. These are senses that are not determined by anything physical, but more by the mind. Candling practitioners also say it helps with developing a second sight and potentially channeling psychic powers.

The ears, just like hands and feet have lots of nerve endings that represent different areas of the body. Ear candling manipulates these nerve endings and can clear them of unwanted energies. It is said that it can also heighten visualization and balance the "chakras" in our bodies. Chakras are the energy centers found in different areas of our being.

This was a small exploration of spiritual ear candling. It

remains an unclear topic with some mysteries although it has been practiced for centuries.

> *Just as a candle cannot burn without fire, men cannot live without a spiritual life...*

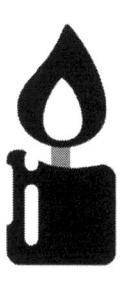

-Buddha-

6
BEST PRACTICES

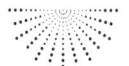

*E*ar candling is a folk medicine where the aim of the practice is to reduce the impurities from within an individual. This is done by placing one end of a hollow candle in the outer ear canal and lighting the other end. The practice is sometimes called ear coning or auriculotherapy. It is believed that the through the lighting of the candle a soft "vacuum" effect is created. This effect then helps remove impurities from the ear and body.

Critics say that candling is a dangerous practice with no benefits. It should be noted however that performing any home remedy incorrectly can be harmful. Everything should be completed with good sense and so reducing the chance of injury. In this chapter we will look into some best practices regarding candling.

. . .

How to

It is recommended to practice ear candling with a trusted partner. Only experienced candlers should attempt to complete the process by themselves.

What you will need:

- **Candles**
- **Paper plate & Scissors:** These are used to prevent any wax or ashes from falling on the subject. Cut a small "X" in the middle of the plate so that the candle can be put through the plate and fit snuggly.
- **Matches:** To light the candle
- **Water:** As a safety measure while handling the small open flame.

The person undergoing the procedure commonly lays down on their side. The ear that is first receiving treatment should be in clear sight and parallel to the flat surface. All hair should be pushed away from the ear. One end of the "candle" (commonly waxed cloth) is placed in the subject's ear. The candle is generally stuck through a small paper plate or similar protectant to prevent hot wax or ashes from falling on the subject. The free end of the candle not in the subjects ear is lit.

The candle then burns for around 20 minutes. It is common for the procedure to last for a little less than an hour long. It can be accompanied with spiritual calming music and end with a soothing head massage. Many claim the procedure to be quite exotic and strange at first, but then relaxing and refreshing. It is normal to feel some heat during a session and to hear some light crackling.

***Important note:** Individuals with medical and artificial ears or any specialized ear conditions should not practice ear candling. If you suffer from cysts or tumors in the area do not use ear candles. It is also important to read the instructions and labels accompanying ear candles. Individuals with certain allergies should make sure they will not react negatively to the wax of the candles.

As mentioned before, ear candling has its fair share of

critics. They claim the practice has no actual health benefits. The practice has a lot of advocates as well, however. Patients claim reduced pain by their ears, and overall better well being. It is a well debated topic regarding a practice that has been around for centuries. These debates are often inconclusive with home cures and spiritual, alternative medicines.

I encourage you to use common sense if you are interested in trying out the practice of candling. Read all instructions carefully on purchased candles, and whenever you are uncomfortable with anything, simply stop. You must feel at ease at all times and it is okay to get help from someone who has experience.

General Tips

- Always have a partner who can supervise and assist.
- Be cautious with the flame. It is small but it is still an open flame.
- Do not squeeze the candle hard. It is hollow and can break if squeezed too hard.
- Once the candle has burned down to only 6-7 inches remaining remove it and stop the flame. This can be done by placing it in a glass filled with water or by covering it with a wet cloth.

- After the procedure is finished, clean the outside of the ear with a cotton swab (Q-tip). Some drops of natural oils can also be used.
- A massage can be done along the forehead, jaws, cheeks and back of the neck. Be gentle with the head and do not move it around much. It should be a relaxing and gentle massage.

"

If you have knowledge, let others light their candles in it...

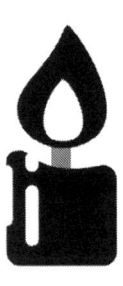

-Margaret Fuller-

7

DOCTORAL THEORIES

*P*hysicians and doctors warn against ear candling. They claim it is an unsafe practice with unregulated devices.

It should be noted that many physicians feel as though more research is required. In terms of healing properties, and from a medical point of view there are better solutions available besides candling.

Medical Issues

The main issue physicians and the FDA have with candling is that it is an unregulated process. It is a good thing to have practices regulated as it ensures safe use. There have been cases where candles have been linked to infections and punctured eardrums. Some unethical practitioners only see candling as a way to make fast money and are not concerned with the safety of patients.

In those situations individuals are at great risk for injury. People have suffered burns and punctures. It relates back to unethical practitioners and not careful applications.

Vacuuming effect

There have been studies completed to determine if candling actually creates a "vacuum" effect. It turns out that there is no negative pressure created by burning an ear candle. This means there is no physical movement of removing impurities from the ears through candling.

It was discovered that there is unfortunately a greater risk of more wax entering the ear than removing the ear.

∽

Ear candle practitioners however continue to believe in the practice. The tradition of candling has been practiced for centuries and it continues to be practiced all over the world today. Individuals feel that there are many spiritual benefits that cannot be explained.

. . .

Even experienced practitioners recommend caution. There are many 'scammers' and they do not help the cause of actual well intentioned individuals. They recommend the use of specific candles.

Physicians recommend individuals to stay away from the procedure. They feel it is fine to use it as decoration and as a pleasant scent, however, it is not something to place inside your ear.

The best candle is understanding...

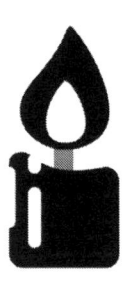

—Welsh Proverbs—

8
OTHER WAYS OF NATURAL EAR CLEANING

*O*ur ears are crucial and sensitive parts of our lives. If we are lucky enough to have properly functioning ears it becomes easy to overlook their importance. It is important to protect them and clean them in a safe manner.

Doctors and specialists recommend for us not to clean them by putting anything inside of our ear canals. In this chapter I wanted to explore some ways to naturally clean one of the more sensitive parts of our bodies.

Natural Cleaning Techniques

Oils

The main culprit we want to get rid of when cleaning the ears is excessive ear wax. A natural solution experts recommend is warmed oils. The kinds of oils suitable are olive oil, baby oil and mineral oil.

A couple drops of warmed oil can be dropped into the ear canal as someone lays on their side. They remain in this position for a couple of seconds so that it can work into the ear wax and weaken it. The oil should be warm, but not hot as this can damage the ear.

Once the oil has been given the time to work in the ear the patient can lean their head to the opposite side so the oil can flow out naturally. It is recommended to have a clean cloth at hand so the oil can be picked up by it.

Next, some clean water can be gently squirted into the ear to remove any wax that didn't seep out yet. One should not rush the process and repeat the above-mentioned steps a couple of times when necessary.

At times it can be helpful to pick up specific ear drops to help with cleaning the ears. They are developed to soften uncomfortable amounts of ear wax. It should be simple to find them at a local pharmacy or drugstore. Please follow the instructions carefully as their application methods may differ.

Heating

Another natural solution is to heat the affected area with a heating pad or pillow. The pad or pillow should be held on the area for about 30 minutes. The warmth from the pillow will loosen up congestion in the ear and with time it will be able to leak out.

A great extra step is to create a salt water mixture and use it to rinse out the ears afterwards. This will both disinfect and clean the area from the buildup.

Relief Technique

A simple way to get a bit of extra relief from pressure in your ear is through working with the connection of your nose and ears. Simply plug your nose shut with your thumb and index finger. Then with your mouth shut try to blow out of your nose. This will blow air through the 'Eustachian' tubes and should relieve some of the pressure in your ears.

Expert opinions

Many specialists advice that the safest solution is to not remove the ear wax at all. This may sound counter productive but the theory is that the body produces ear wax for several reasons. It is how the body naturally protects the area. It stops dirt and infections from traveling deeper into the ear canal. Using a cotton swab may sound appealing at first but actually it is just likely that you are pushing ear wax deeper down your ear canal. This can eventually lead to difficulties hearing because of compressing built up ear wax. Or even worse, puncturing the eardrum.

It can be recommended to only remove ear wax when it is truly excessive and causes loss of hearing. The body will regulate the amount of ear wax it should produce if left alone. If you are experiencing irregular amounts or earwax or discolorations, then it is best to visit a specialist. They will be able to tell if there is a bigger issue that may need to be handled.

Burn not thy fingers to snuff another man's candle...

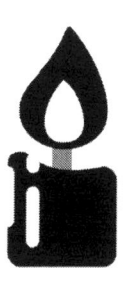

-James Howell-

AFTERWORD

Ear candling is not an easy topic to tackle. On the one hand it is a respected tradition that has been around for centuries, on the other it is a highly controversial procedure. My aim was to provide an unbiased insight on the topic. We looked at the history, techniques, traditions and critiques surrounding ear candling.

I have grown to respect the various views on the topic. I understand concerns physicians may have, yet I have a deep admiration for the spiritual guidance and well being it provides others. I want to encourage you to continue finding out more about ear candling if it interests you. It is always recommended to speak to a doctor before using any treatment. Be safe with your hearing and your body...

> A good teacher is like a candle – it consumes itself to light the way for others...

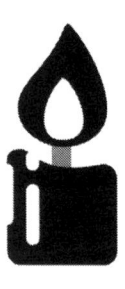

―Mustafa Kemal Ataturk―

THANK YOU

Thank you for reading this book, I hope you enjoyed!

If you found the information provided useful, I would truly appreciate you leaving a review. Your honest opinion will make it easier for other readers to make a good purchasing decision. You will also be helping me compete with big publishing companies who have large advertising budgets and get hundreds of reviews. Thank you for your considerations and have an awesome day!

RESOURCES PAGE

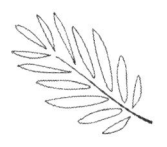

Besides my own knowledge and experiences, I used the following awesome sources to create this book:

Berger, Alan S. "The Interconnected World of the Ear, Nose, and Throat." *BergerHenry ENT Specialty Group*, 17 Apr. 2018, www.bergerhenryent.com/the-interconnected-world-of-the-ear-nose-throat/.

Hoffman, Matthew. "What Are the Sinuses? Pictures of Nasal Cavities." *WebMD*, WebMD, www.webmd.com/allergies/picture-of-the-sinuses#1.

N/A, N/A. "Hopi Ear Candling: Inspirational Therapies: Glenrothes, Fife." *Inspirational Therapies*, www.inspirationaltherapies.co.uk/therapies/hopi-ear-candling/.

N/A. "Blocked and Clogged Ears: 10 Tips for Unclogging

& Pressure Relief." *WebMD*, WebMD, www.webmd.com/allergies/stuffy-ears-sinuses#1.

N/A. "Ear, Nose, and Throat Facts." *Department of Otolaryngology Head and Neck Surgery*, www.entcolumbia.org/staywell/document.php?id=33636.

N/A. "Hopi Ear Candling." *Wai Chung Yoga*, waichungyoga.com/hopi-ear-candle/.

Traynor, Robert. "Ear Candling to Remove Wax: Is It Real or a Hoax?" *Hearing International*, 18 Mar. 2019, hearinghealthmatters.org/hearinginternational/2013/ear-candling-hoax-or-reality/.

Printed in Poland
by Amazon Fulfillment
Poland Sp. z o.o., Wrocław